Mediterranean Diet

Step By Step Guide And Proven Recipes For Smart Eating And Weight Loss

Introduction

I want to thank you and congratulate you for purchasing the book, *"Mediterranean Diet – Step By Step Guide And Proven Recipes For Smart Eating And Weight Loss"*.

This book contains proven steps and strategies on how to follow the Mediterranean diet properly, not just for the best results in weight loss but for optimum health too.

The Mediterranean diet is, without a doubt, the healthiest diet on earth. It is also one of the oldest and, as such, is proven to work. I will be explaining the principles of the Mediterranean diet to you in simple and easy to understand terms, along with tips on how to do the diet properly and how not to do it. I will also give you an easy reference list of the foods you can eat and those that you should avoid. Finally, I will finish off with some delicious recipes for you to try; I promise that, once you have tried them, you won't want to go back to your old way of eating! I will be showing you some wonderful breakfasts, a choice of soups and salads, main courses, a few delicious desserts and even some easy to prepare snacks.

Thanks again for purchasing this book, I hope you enjoy it!

Bonus: FREE Report Reveals The Secrets To Lose Weight

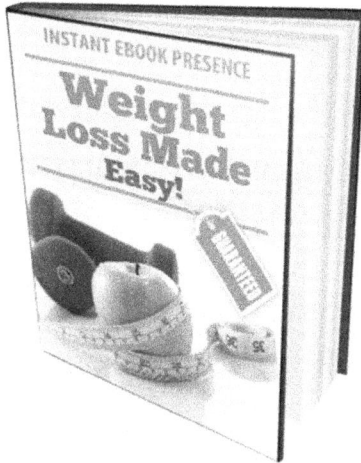

Weight loss doesn't happen from dieting only. Diets are short term solutions to shed extra weight. Diets do not work in the long term because people hate being on a diet (it's ok, you can admit that here). The only long term solution for permanent weight loss is to create new eating habits. This doesn't mean that chocolate will never pass your lips again, but it does mean looking after yourself and watching what you eat...

You can lose weight when you have the right reasons and motivation, and a part of this guide is to help you to find the motivation you need to change your weight...

Click Here to Get This Guid For FREE

Table Of Content

Chapter 1: How Will the Mediterranean Diet Benefit You?

For many people, foods like lasagna, gyros, pizza, rack of lamb and loaves of white bread are what makes up the Mediterranean diet, most likely because this is what they eat when they visit a Mediterranean country. We tend to think of long, wine filled lunches, with many courses and this is what the original Mediterranean diet was like. However, the last 50 years or so have seen a huge change; Mediterranean meals have been pumped full of unhealthy fat and calories, pushing aside the traditional foods of the region. What used to be a very healthy and cheap way of eating is now firmly associated with a range of different diseases – obesity, heart disease, mood disorders, diabetes, and much more besides. And that's not to mention the fact that what used to be a healthy way of eating is now unhealthy and filled with heavy fatty dishes, at least for the tourist aspects. For the people who live in the Mediterranean, things are different.

When World War II had concluded, Ansel Keys from the Mayo Clinic studied the diets of around 13,000 men. All of them were middle-aged and they lived across the US, Italy, Japan, Greece, Finland, The Netherlands, and Yugoslavia. His conclusions were a revelation – American men, very well-fed, showed much higher heart disease rates than in any other country that had been struck by the rations and deprivations that took place during the war. The poorest people in Key's study were those men who lived on the Greek Island of Crete and they had, without any doubt, the best heart health of any of those studied. This was down to the physical work they did and their food pyramid, somewhat unique compared to the rest of the world.

The food pyramid for the Mediterranean diet is based on the diet traditions from the 1960's in Greece, Crete, and Southern Italy. This was a time when chronic disease was at its lowest level in these countries and life expectancy was much higher than anywhere in the world, despite having a very limited access to medical services. Their diet consisted of homegrown and fresh food but it wasn't just that – the Mediterranean people exercise daily, they share their meals with others and they fully appreciate the pleasure of eating the food they have.

8 Benefits of A Mediterranean Diet

The Mediterranean diet is loaded with benefits, not least the delicious foods and wine that you get to enjoy on a daily basis. These are the 8 main benefits of the diet:

1. Low Sugar and Low in Processed Foods

The Mediterranean diet consists mainly of natural foods and ingredients, such as legumes, olives oil, vegetables, fruits, unrefined cereals, and small amounts of animal products (preferably local sourced and organic). In contrast to a typical Western diet, it has little sugar in it and virtually free from GMO or other artificial ingredients, such as HFCS (high-fructose corn syrup). If you have a sweet tooth, the Mediterranean diet provides amply, with fruits, and homemade desserts that use honey for natural sweetness.

Aside from vegetation-based foods, the diet also has another staple – local caught fresh fish and small amounts of cheeses and yogurts made from sheep, cow, or goat milk. These provide an excellent and healthy way to get healthy fats and healthy cholesterol into your diet. Sardines, anchovies, and other similar fish are central to the diet and are eaten more than meat products. While the people of the Mediterranean are not vegetarian, the diet consists of small amounts only of meats and other heavier foods, opting instead for lighter and healthier meals that include fish. This is highly beneficial for those who want to shed some weight and improve their health in terms of heart health, cholesterol, and their intake of omega-3 fatty acids.

2. Lose Weight Healthily

The Mediterranean diet promotes healthy weight loss without leaving you hungry and helps you to maintain your new weight in a realistic and sustainable way for the rest of your life. The Mediterranean diet enjoys huge success around the whole world with people who want to lose weight as is helps you to reduce your intake of fat in a natural and easy way, thanks to the amount of nutrient-dense foods that you eat.

The Mediterranean diet is not a strict one and is open to a small measure of interpretation. Some people prefer to cut their carbs, their proteins or stay somewhere in the middle and that can be done on this diet as it focuses on consuming a good amount of healthy fat while keeping levels of carbohydrate intake low and increasing the intake of healthy proteins. If you prefer to eat more meat than legumes, that is fine because you will still lose weight without any sense of deprivation, eating a higher level of seafood and high quality dairy. All of these also provide other benefits in the form of probiotics and omeaga-3s.

Grass fed meats, dairy products, and wild caught fish contain good amounts of fatty acids that are essential to the working of the human body. They help you to feel fuller for longer, keep your blood sugar levels down and improve your energy and mood. If you prefer to eat more of a plant-based diet, you can get the same results with legumes and healthy whole grains, particularly those that have been soaked and sprouted.

3. Improves Your Heart Health

Research has shown that those who adhere to the Mediterranean diet, consuming plenty of omega-3 foods and monounsaturated fats, have a much lower mortality rate from heart disease. A diet that is rich in ALA (alpha-linolenic acid) found in olive oil, such as the Mediterranean diet, has been shown to have very high protective levels and can decrease the risk of death from cardiac arrest by up to 30% and the risk of sudden cardiac death by up to 45%.

Research carried out at the Warwick Medical School on blood pressure showed that when the levels were compared between those who ate a diet high in extra-virgin olive oil and those who consumed more sunflower oil, those on the olive oil had significantly lower blood pressure. This is because olive oil increases the bioavailability of nitric oxide and keeps your arteries clearer and more dilated.

4. Helps to Fight off Some Cancers

The European Journal of Cancer Prevention says that "the biological mechanisms for cancer prevention associated with the Mediterranean diet have been related to the favorable effect of a balanced ratio of omega-6 and omega-3 essential fatty acids and high amounts of fiber, antioxidants and polyphenols found in fruit, vegetables, olive oil and wine."

To quantify that, plant foods, in particular vegetables and fruits, are the basis of the Mediterranean diet and it is these

4

foods that help to fight off cancer in virtually every single way. They do this because they are full of antioxidants, they protect your DNA from becoming damaged, they stop cells from mutating and they lower inflammation, as well as slowing down the growth of tumors. There are a lot of studies that point to olive oil consumption as being a natural cure for cancer and for decreasing the risk of bowel and colon cancer. It could be that it has a protective effect on cancer cell development because of its propensity for reducing inflammation and reducing oxidative stress. It also helps to promote a healthy weight and better blood sugar balance.

5. Can Help to Treat or Prevent Diabetes

There is evidence to suggest that the Mediterranean diet helps to fight off inflammatory diseases, including type 2 diabetes and metabolic syndrome. The main reason why the Mediterranean diet is successful at preventing these diseases is because it controls insulin production. Insulin is a hormone that controls your blood sugar, and in many diets, is responsible for weight gain and a struggle to lose it, no matter how many diets we undertake.

By controlling blood sugar levels with the right balance of healthy whole foods, the body is able to burn off fat better and provide more energy. A diet that is low in sugar and high in fresh foods and healthy fats is a natural cure for diabetes. The American Heart Association says that the Mediterranean diet is actually higher in fat than a normal American diet but it is lower in levels of saturated fat. The diet is normally a ratio of about 40% complex carbohydrate, 30-40% healthy fat, and 20-30% high quality protein. This is the ideal balance for keeping your hunger and weight eves under control and for keeping the body in hormonal homeostasis, thus normalizing insulin levels.

The sugar in the diet comes mainly from wine, fruit, and the odd local dessert. Most people tend to drink water, coffee, and red wine, rather than the popular sodas and fizzy drinks consumed across the Western world as a whole. Some versions of the Mediterranean diet do contain carbohydrates in the form of pasta and bread but the activity levels and low sugar consumption of the diet also mean that resistance to insulin is rare, cutting out the dips and spikes in blood sugar that contribute towards diabetes.

Most people in the Mediterranean will eat a well-balanced breakfast within 2 hours of waking up. This helps to balance off their blood sugar when it as its lowest point. They will eat three filling meals a day, full of healthy fiber and fats and tend to have their largest meal at midday, rather than at night. Opposite to this is the standard American diet, which is composed of no breakfast, snacks throughout the day on high carbohydrate and high sugar foods and eating large meals at night when they are not active.

6. Help to Improve Mood and Cognitive Function

Studies show that the Mediterranean diet can help to treat diseases such as Parkinson's, Alzheimer's and dementia and can also slow the onset of these diseases. Cognitive disease happens when there are insufficient levels of dopamine in the brain – this is an important chemical for the proper movement of the body, thought processing and regulating moods.

Healthy fats, like those found in nuts and olive oil, plus the anti-inflammatory properties of the copious amounts of vegetables and fruits, are well known to help fight off age-related cognitive disorders. They help to counteract the harmful effects of exposure to free radicals and toxicity, food allergies and inflammation, all of which contribute towards an impairment in brain function. Studies show that people who adhere to the Mediterranean diet display lower rates of Alzheimer's than in any other diet. Adding probiotics, such as those found in kefir and yogurt, also help to promote a healthy gut, which, as we know, is vital for improving mood and memory disorders.

7. Can Help to Prolong Life Expectancy

Diets that are high in fresh plant-based foods and healthy fat have been shown to be the best combination for longevity. That main fat source in the Mediterranean diet is monounsaturated fat and is found in nuts and olive oil. Research over the years has shown that this is the best type of fat for lowering the risk of heart disease, depression, cancer, Alzheimer's disease, cognitive decline, inflammatory disease and much more besides. These diseases are the leading causes, in the developed nations, of death.

The Lyon Diet Heart Study looked at those who had suffered heart attacks between 1988 and 1992. The participants of the study were asked to either follow a Mediterranean type diet or follow a standard diet for the post-heart attack, which reduced saturated fat significantly. After 4 years, the results showed that those who followed the Mediterranean diet had 70% less heart disease, three times the risk-reduction that is achieved through statins, the prescription drug for lowering cholesterol. They also showed 45% less risk of all-cause death than those on the standard post-heart attack diet.

One thing that stood out among the results was that there was little change in levels of cholesterol which just shows that, contrary to what we are told, there is far more to heart disease than high cholesterol.

8. Helps you Relax

One last factor is that the Mediterranean diet encourages people to sleep better, spend more time in nature and bond with other people over a god healthy home-cooked meal. These are all great ways to lower stress levels, which, in turn, lowers inflammation. On the whole, people in the Mediterranean tend to spend more time outside and enjoy their meals with family and friends in a relaxed setting. They also set time aside to practice their hobbies, dance, laugh, enjoy the garden, and generally enjoy themselves.

Chapter 2: The Ten Commandments of the Mediterranean Diet

While we already know what the benefits of the Mediterranean diet are, actually adopting the proper Mediterranean way of eating is not quite as simple as you may believe, certainly not the way many cookbooks would have you believe. Yes, there are plenty of recipes that are promoted as being Mediterranean but they may not be the ones that are the best for us, according to the research. In many cases, these are dishes that are masquerading as the fare that we believe to be Mediterranean.

The main reason for this is because many cookery books seem to focus on desserts and festive foods from particular regions. We tend to think of foods like viros, souvlaki, and other meat-filled dishes but the real Mediterranean diet, the true one that was made famous back in the 1960's is more of a vegetarian based diet. It was called the "poor man's diet: because there wasn't much meat. More fish was included because it was more available but the main diet was legumes and plant foods, healthy sources of protein.

Casseroles were served which would contain little meat but plenty of vegetables such as peas, artichokes, carrots, and zucchini, and would always be accompanied by a side salad. On average a person would consume half a kilo each of vegetables and fruit per day.

To help you get the idea of what the diet actually involves, Dr. Catherine Itsopoulos, accredited practicing dietician, has come up with 10 commandments:

- Aim to consume around 60 ml of olive oil per day, using it as your main source of added fat

- Eat vegetables with every single meal, aiming for 100g of tomato, 100g of leafy greens and 200g of other vegetables per day.

- Eat at least two meals containing 250g of legumes each week

- Eat two servings of fish per week as a minimum guide. Each serving should be 150-200g and you should include oily fish, such as salmon, trevalla, sardines, mackerel, and gemfish. Canned tuna doesn't contain such high levels of omega-3 as tuna fillet, but is still a decent choice

- Eat meat, such as lamb, beef, pork, and chicken no more than a couple of times per week and make the portions small, bulking up with vegetables.

- Eat fresh fruit every single day and eat dried nuts and dried fruits for dessert or snacks

- Consume about 200g of yogurt every day and around 30-40g of cheese per day

- Make sure you include whole grain cereals and bread with your meals – aim for a consumption of about 3 or 4 slices of whole grain bread per day

- Drink red wine in moderation – a standard drink every day, about 100 ml. Only drink with meals and never over-indulge Try to keep away from alcohol entirely for two days of the week.

- Sweets and sugary drinks should only be consumed for special occasions and always in moderation.

Chapter 3: Busting the Mediterranean Diet Myths

There are plenty of benefits to the Mediterranean diet and no doubt you have heard loads of things about it. Not everything you read or hear is necessarily true, though, in particular, the claims that you can eat vast meals of rich food and knock back gallons of red wine. In this chapter, I am going to bust some of those myths that you may have heard about the Mediterranean diet:

1. Everyone who lies in the Mediterranean is healthy

The Mediterranean covers a vast amount of land and coast, including Greece, Turkey, Morocco, Italy, France, even parts of North Africa and not every region follows the same eating habits. For example, in northern Italy, they use more butter and lard in their cooking, consuming larger amounts of saturated fats, whereas, in southern Italy, they tend to use more olive oil. The basis for the Mediterranean diet for health is inspired by Greece, Crete, Morocco, southern Italy, and Spain.

2. You can eat vast amounts of cheese

Too much cheese does nothing more than pile on the pounds, high in calories and in saturated fat. While consumption of cheese is a Mediterranean practice, it is only in moderation and they tend to go for stronger cheeses, like goat cheese or feta. This can give you the flavor without eating a large amount of cheese.

3. Drinking copious amounts of red wine is good for your heart

While red wine does have health benefits, specifically for the heart, moderation is the real key. If you regularly drink more than a couple of glasses of wine, it can actually cause damage to your heart. One glass per day with a meal is the recommended amount for heart health.

4. It's fine to eat big portions of pasta with bread

Many people tend to think of Italian cooking, especially pasta when they think of the Mediterranean. Pasta needs bread otherwise you can't soak the sauce up. Yes, Italians do eat a lot of pasta but not in huge portions, the way Americans do. Mediterranean portions are typically side dishes and are around ½ to 1 cup. It is never served as a dish on its own and is generally accompanied by meat, salads, and vegetables. One slice of bread may also be consumed

5. You don't need to exercise on the Mediterranean diet

You do but you don't need to take out an expensive gym membership. The traditional Mediterranean lifestyle involves physical work and walking instead of driving. If you don't live a life where you can get out in the garden each day or walk instead of driving, then you will need to find alternative means of exercising every day.

6. Mediterranean people can eat huge meals and they never put on weight

This is technically not true. While Mediterranean people do tend to eat large meals, these are made up of several smaller dishes, usually low calorie, rather than one huge serving. They eat lots of raw and cooked vegetables, and small portions of legumes, meat, and grains. What is important is how the meal is made up, not how small or large it is. You can't eat whatever you want and expect to lose weight; it comes down to balance.

7. The Mediterranean diet is expensive

If you use legumes, beans and lentils as your main protein source and you stick to mainly whole grains and plants, the Mediterranean diet works out much cheaper than serving up processed and packaged foods.

8. The Mediterranean Diet is only based on food

While the food is a very big part of the Mediterranean diet, we must forget the other things that go into making up their way of life. When they eat, it isn't a rushed meal and it isn't in front of the TV; instead, they eat a leisurely meal with lots of company and this could be just as important as what you eat. Factor in the physical wok they do on a daily basis and the fact that they walk wherever they can, and you can see that this isn't just about the food.

9. All vegetable oils are good for you and they are all the same

If only things were that simple! There are actually two basic unsaturated vegetable oils – the traditional cold-pressed variety, such as peanut and extra-virgin olive oil that are high in healthy monounsaturated fats and made without heat or chemicals to extract the oils. The second are those that are processed in a modern way, like the sunflower, corn, soybean, cottonseed, canola, vegetable, and safflower oils. These are manufactured industrially from GM crops and use toxic solvents and high heat to get the oil out of the seeds. This kind of processing can damage the oil and turn the healthy fatty acids into trans fats, the most dangerous of all.

They also contain a high level of omega-6, which upsets the omega 6 to 3 ratio that is vital for health.

Chapter 4: What You Should Be Eating (And What to Avoid)

There really isn't any right or wrong way to do the Mediterranean diet, simply because the Mediterranean is made up of so many countries that all eat differently. The basics of the diet for health are as follows but bear in mind that this is open to interpretation depending on your own circumstances, preferences, and needs.

What to Eat

Fish and Poultry

Eat two servings per week instead of red meat, which is limited to no more than 16 oz. a month.

- Turkey
- Chicken
- Shrimp
- Oysters
- Salmon
- Mackerel
- Squid
- Mussels
- Lobster
- Tuna
- Tilapia
- Founder
- Salmon

Healthy Fats

Stick to olive oil on the whole and canola on occasion. Olive oil is used as a seasoning and as a preparation food.

Vegetables and Fruits

Consume in abundance

- Artichokes
- Celery
- Eggplant
- Broccoli
- Peas
- Onions
- Peppers
- Lettuce
- Sweet potatoes
- Mushrooms
- Tomatoes
- Apples
- Melons
- Grapefruit
- Peaches
- Dates
- Strawberries
- Cherries

- Peaches

Dairy

Eat low to moderate amounts of milk, cheese, and yogurt but do use low or fat-free versions and try, where possible to eat those made by locally produced cow, sheep, and goat milk.

Grains

Eat whole grains only:

- wheat
- bulgar
- rice
- couscous
- barley
- spelt

Beverages

- One glass of red wine per day with a meal.
- Avoid sugary soft drinks, fruit juices, drink a little coffee and lots of water

Nuts

Eat in moderation and try to stick to nuts that grow on trees, like almonds, walnuts, and pecans. Choose unsalted nuts and do not eat those that have been candied

This list is clearly not exhaustive because there are so many different foods available across the Mediterranean. The rule of thumb is lots of fresh, local, and organic fruits and vegetables and where you eat dairy, meat or fish, opt for free range or wild-caught versions rather than those packaged in supermarkets

At all costs, avoid packaged and processed foods, sunflower and vegetable oils, margarine, anything with HCFS, added sugars and trans fats. Do read packet labels carefully

Just How Important is Olive Oil?

Virtually every nutritionist and researcher will attribute some of the health benefits of the diet to the generous amounts of olive oil that are used in every meal. Olives are, perhaps, one of the most ancient of foods, and olive trees have been growing across the Mediterranean since 3000 BC.

Olive oil is one of the elite foods containing healthy omega-3 fatty acids, joining the likes of walnuts and salmon. The health benefits of olive oil are firmly backed up by so much research that even the FDA has allowed the labels on bottles of olive oil to contain a health claim. Limited research, certainly not conclusive, suggests that consuming 2 tablespoons of olive oil every day is enough to cut the risk of heart disease because of the monounsaturated fat it contains. To achieve this, however, it is not enough to consume the olive oil; it has to be used to replace a similar level of saturated fat and not in addition to it.

So, what does olive oil, the mainstay of the Mediterranean diet, contain that makes it so good for you?

For a start, it is high in phenols, which are antioxidants that can fight damage caused by free radicals and lower inflammation. Olive oil is mainly monounsaturated fatty acids, with the most important of these being oleic acid. This is known to be healthy for the heart in several ways, especially when you compare it to hydrogenated, trans or refined fats and oils.

Olive oil is even a step above many of the grain-based carbohydrates when it comes to heart health. For example, the high levels of monounsaturated fats lower LDL cholesterol while raising HDL and reducing triglycerides far more effectively than a carb heavy diet does.

A beneficial amount of olive oil to consume on a daily basis is up to four tablespoons per day but this will depend on your caloric requirements. What you do have to remember is that there is more than one type of olive oil and this will have an effect. Many of the commercial manufacturers are trying to get on the olive oil health bandwagon by producing fake oil. These are nothing more than bad imitations that are actually bad for your health. The reason for this is because they are not harvested properly and are most certainly not processed in the right way and this can not only kill off some of the more delicate nutrients, it can also turn the fatty acids toxic or rancid.

To get the right oils, look for those that are labeled as cold-pressed and extra-virgin. Olive oil is, quite possibly, the most unique oil in that it can be consumed in its crude form without the need or any processing. You could actually press a bucket of olives and enjoy the oils as it comes.

One more tip about olive oil; if you are not sure if you have bought the real thing, put it in the freezer. True olive oil will NOT freeze so if it does its fake. Do make sure you purchase oil in dark glass bottles and do make sure the oil is made in the same region as the olives are harvested.

How to Follow the Mediterranean Diet at Restaurants

Most restaurant meals can be made suitable for the Mediterranean diet:

- Order seafood or fish for your main dish

- Ask them to use extra virgin olive oil for any fried foods

- Only consume whole grain bread and use olive oil rather than butter

Chapter 5: A Quick Start Guide to the Mediterranean Diet

Making the change is the hardest part about doing the Mediterranean diet but, to help you out, here are some simple guidelines and suggestions to help you get started:

- Swap vegetable oil for olive oil for sautéing

- Have a salad as a starter or side, have fruit as snacks and increase your vegetable intake

- Forget the refined pasta, bread, and rice; choose whole grain versions instead

- Cut red meat down by substituting 2 meals per week with fish

- Eat more dairy products, such as cheese, milk, and yogurt. Go for plain yogurt that you can dress up with nuts, fruit, and honey. Enjoy natural cheeses made from sheep, cow, and goat milk, locally produced. Whole milk products are linked to lower levels of body fat and a lower risk of obesity, mostly because these products make you feel fuller for longer.

- Eat more vegetables. Try eating a plate of tomatoes sliced up with olive oil and feta cheese. Layer peppers and mushrooms on your pizza instead of pepperoni and sausage. Eat more salad, homemade soups, and platters of crudités to get more vegetables into your diet

- You must change how you see meat – it is not a big part of the diet and, where you do eat it, you should opt for the grass-fed versions instead of that which has been industrially raised. Add strips of organic chicken to a salad and add a little amount of meat to a whole-wheat pasta dish

- Never miss breakfast. Start the day the right way with whole grains, fruit and any other food rich in fiber that keeps you satiated for longer

- Make sure you eat a seafood dish twice a week. The best ones, those rich in omega-3 fatty acids, are the salmon, tuna, black cod, herring, sardines, oysters, mussels, and clams.

- Have a vegetarian meal once a week, building your meal up around vegetables, whole grains, and beans. When you get used to it, increase to twice a week.

- Always use the good fats in your meals. Go for the extra virgin olive oil, avocado, olives and sunflower seeds as well as nuts in moderation

- If you have a sweet tooth, swap the cakes and ice cream for fresh fruit like fresh figs with honey, strawberries, apples and grapes, all locally grown produce.

Mercury in Fish

We all know that fish has massive health benefits but there are also the concerns over pollutants, such as traces of the mercury, a toxic heavy metal. This is found in just about all fish and shellfish and you need to be able to make the right and the safest choices when you buy fish.

The rule of thumb is that, the larger the fish, the higher the concentration of pollutants and mercury. Try to avoid the largest fish, such as king mackerel, shark, tilefish, and swordfish.

You should be able to safely consume around 12 oz. of cooked seafood per week, split into 2 portions of 6 oz. each

If you are eating locally caught seafood, pay attention to any advisories about what is safe to eat and what you should avoid

If you are pregnant or nursing a child, or are a child under the age of 12, go for fish that have the lower levels of mercury, such as canned light tuna, shrimp, pollock, salmon, and catfish. If you eat Albacore tuna, be aware that it has a higher level of mercury and, as such, you should eat no more than 6 oz. per week

Ideas for Alternative Foods

You should start slowly, swapping foods out gradually to get yourself used to the Mediterranean diet. Try these delicious food swaps:

Instead of:	Try This:
Pretzels, chips, crackers with ranch dip	Broccoli, celery, carrots with salsa
White rice and a stir-fried meat	Quinoa with some stir-fried vegetables
Sandwiches made with white bread/rolls	Healthy fillings in whole-wheat tortillas
Ice cream	Puddings made with milk
Toast for breakfast	Plain yogurt with fruit and honey

Now that you know the basics of the Mediterranean diet, it's time to look at some recipes so that you can see just how satisfying the diet is.

Chapter 6: Breakfast

Yogurt with Honey and Apricots

Preparation time: 5 minutes

Serves 6

Ingredients

- 1 cup of Greek yogurt, low fat
- 2 tbsp. organic honey
- ½ tsp vanilla extract
- 9 fresh apricots, cut in half lengthways

Instructions

1. Whisk the yogurt together with the vanilla and honey
2. Arrange the apricots in bowls and spoon the yogurt mixture over the top
3. Serve straight away or chill first

Mediterranean Stuffed Tomatoes

Preparation time: 10 minutes

Cooking time: 5 minutes

Serves 1

Ingredients:

- 2 large tomatoes
- ½ cup garlic croutons, pre-packaged or homemade
- ¼ cup goat cheese, crumbled
- ¼ cup Kalamata olives, pitted and sliced
- 2 tbsp. Italian salad dressing or low fat vinaigrette
- 2 tbsp. fresh chopped basil or thyme

Instructions:

1. Preheat the broiler
2. Slice the tomatoes in half crossways
3. Discard the seeds, using your finger to push them out
4. Use a small knife to remove the pulp – you should be left with two shells
5. Chop up the pulp and put it into a medium bowl
6. Put the tomato shells onto a paper towel, cut side down and leave to drain for 5 minutes
7. Add the olives, croutons, goats cheese and herbs in the bowl with the tomato pulp and mix together; add the dressing and combine well

8. Spoon the mixture into the hollowed-out tomato shells

9. Place them on a baking tray or a broiler pan and broil for about 5 minutes. They should be 4 or 5 inches away from the heat and the cheese should be melted

10. Serve straightaway

Breakfast Couscous

Preparation time: 20 minutes

Cooking time: 5 minutes

Serves 4

Ingredients:

- 3 cups low fat milk, 1%
- 1 cinnamon stick, about 2 inches in length
- 1 cup whole wheat couscous, uncooked
- ¼ cup dried currants
- ½ cup dried chopped apricots
- 6 tsp dark brown soft sugar
- ¼ tsp salt
- 4 tsp melted butter

Instructions:

1. Place the milk into a large pan and heat with the cinnamon stick for 3 minutes over a medium-high heat. Do not allow to boil, just let bubbles begin to form around the edge of the milk

2. Take the milk from the heat and add the couscous, fruit, salt, and 4 tsp of sugar. Mix together well and cover; leave to stand for 15 minutes

3. Take the cinnamon stick out and divide the mixture between 4 bowls

4. Top off with 1 tsp of melted butter and ½ tsp sugar' serve straightaway

Greek Yogurt with Honey, Oats, and Mixed Berries

Preparation time: 5 minutes

Serves 1

Ingredients:

- ¼ Greek yogurt, full fat
- ¼ cup fresh or frozen mixed berries
- ¼ cup oats
- Small handful of fresh walnuts
- Honey

Instructions:

1. Put the berries into a bowl. If they are frozen, microwave for 30 seconds
2. Add the yogurt, walnuts, and oats
3. Mix gently and drizzle honey over the top
4. Serve straightaway or chill first

Avocado Toast

Preparation time: 5 minutes

Cooking time: 5 minutes

Serves 2

Ingredients:

- 2 avocados, small and ripe, pitted, and peeled
- ¾ cup crumbled feta cheese
- 2 tbsp. fresh chopped mint, plus a little extra for garnishing
- 4 slices wholegrain rye bread
- Squeeze of lemon juice

Instructions:

1. Roughly mash the avocado with a fork in a medium bowl
2. Add the mint and mix in with a squeeze of lemon juice, mashing until combined
3. Season with salt and pepper
4. Toast the bread and spoon the avocado mixture over the toast
5. Top off with feta and serve with a garnish of fresh mint

For a larger meal, add some shaved ham or a poached egg

Frittata

Preparation time: 10 minutes

Cooking time 25 minutes

Serves 6

Ingredients:

- 1 cup chopped onion
- 2 cloves minced garlic
- 3 tbsp. extra virgin olive oil
- 8 beaten eggs
- ¼ cup light cream, milk or half and half
- ½ cup feta, crumbled
- ½ cup bottled roasted red pepper, chopped
- ½ cup Kalamata or other olives, pitted
- ¼ cup fresh slivered basil
- 1/8 tsp ground black pepper
- ½ cup garlic and onion croutons, crushed coarsely
- 2 tbsp. parmesan cheese, shredded finely
- Fresh basil leaves for garnish

Instructions:

1. Preheat your broiler
2. In a broiler-proof pan or skillet, heat the oil and cook the garlic and onion for about 2 minutes, or until the onion is tender

3. Mix the beaten eggs with the milk in a separate bowl

4. Stir in the peppers, feta, olives, black pepper, and basil

5. Pour the mixture over the onions and cook until set, running a spatula around the edge to lift the mixture as it sets. This ensures that all the mixture is cooked

6. Mix the croutons with 1 tbsp. oil. And the cheese and sprinkle it over the frittata mixture

7. Broil about 4 inches away from the heat until the crumbs have turned golden and the top is set firmly

8. Cut into wedges and serve with fresh basil leaves

Chapter 7: Soups

Fish Soup

Preparation time: 15 minutes

Cooking time: 30 minutes

Serves 4

Ingredients:

- 1 lb. live mussels
- 1 lb. live clams
- 1 lb. white fish cut into ½ inch slices – Monkfish is a good one
- 1 lb. uncooked prawns or shrimps with shells on
- 4 small calamari (squid)
- 4 finely chopped garlic cloves
- ½ liter fish stock OR one fish stock cube
- 8 ½ oz dry white wine
- 1 small red pepper, roasted and diced finely
- Juice from ½ a lemon
- 1 bunch chopped parsley
- 1 tsp turmeric powder
- 1 tsp corn flour or corn starch
- Salt and pepper for seasoning

Instructions:

1. Put the wine and stock into a large pan and heat; add the mussels and cook until they open. Remove any that don't open and if you don't use all of the mussels, freeze them on the half shell

2. Remove the opened mussels and add the clams to the liquid

3. Cook until they open, discarding any that don't

4. Remove the clams and add shrimp or prawns to the liquid, cooking until pink. These are for garnish so don't use too many

5. Remove the cooked prawns and set aside

6. Shell the remainder of the prawns

7. Slice the squid into ½ inch rounds and fry the squid and prawns in olive oil with the garlic until cooked through

8. Strain the liquid using a fine sieve and return it to the pan

9. Add the white fish and cook over a medium heat, stirring until cooked

10. Add the turmeric, lemon juice, corn flour and most of the parsley; bring back to a simmer

11. Add the clams, shrimp, and squid back to the liquid and heat through

12. Arrange the mussels and the first lot of prawns on soup plates and pour the soup over the top

13. Sprinkle the rest of the parsley over the top and serve hot

Tomato Soup

Preparation time: 10 minutes

Cooking time: 15 minutes

Serves 4

Ingredients:

The Soup

- 2 cans Italian plum tomatoes, chopped (16 oz. cans) OR use the same weight of fresh skinned and chopped tomatoes
- 32 oz. vegetable stock
- 1 tsp tomato puree
- 1 rough chopped medium onion
- 2 bashed garlic cloves
- 1 tsp sugar
- 1 tsp dried basil
- Small handful fresh basil leaves
- Half a lemon, juiced
- 4 oz. Greek yogurt
- Salt and pepper for seasoning

The Croutons

1. 12 thin slices of a stale baguette, whole meal
2. Olive oil
3. 1 oz. parmesan cheese, fresh grated

Instructions:

1. Heat a little olive oil and sauté the onion; do not let it brown

2. Add the garlic, turn down the heat and sauté for a few minutes

3. Add the basil, tomato, sugar, and the stock and bring up to the boil

4. While it cooks, sprinkle the bread slices with olive oil and top off with the grated cheese; grill until golden

5. Allow the soup to boil gently for a minute or 2 and then use a stick blender to blend it in the pan

6. Spoon into bowls and stop off with the croutons and fresh basil leaves

Sweet Potato Soup

Preparation time: 10 minutes

Cooking time: 40 minutes

Serves 4-6

Instructions:

- 2 tbsp. extra virgin olive oil
- 1 large chopped onion
- 2 lb. sweet potato, peeled and chopped into medium size pieces
- ½ tsp ground cumin
- ¼ tsp ground chili
- ¼ tsp ground cinnamon
- ½ tsp ground coriander
- ¼ tsp salt
- A little more than 2 cups chicken stock
- Low fat crème Fraiche for garnish
- Fresh chopped coriander or parsley for garnish

Instructions:

1. Heat the olive oil over a high heat and sauté the onion until it begins to color
2. Turn the heat to medium and sauté the garlic for a few minutes, stirring well
3. Add the sweet potato to the pan and sauté for a few minutes

4. Add the spices and salt, stir well, and cook for 2 minutes

5. Pour the stock in, increase the heat and bring up to the boil; give it one more stir and cover the pan

6. Reduce the heat and simmer for 2 minutes until the potato has softened

7. Take the pan off the heat and use a hand blender to blend until smooth

8. If the soup is too thick, add a little stock or water

9. Season to taste and serve in warm bowls.

10. Swirl the crème Fraiche through the soup and garnish with the parsley or coriander

Seafood Bisque

Preparation time: 20 minutes

Cooking time: 60 minutes

Serves 4

Ingredients:

The Soup

- 1 lb. uncooked, shell-on shrimp or prawns – peeled and heads removed (reserve for the stock)
- 8 oz. white fish, chopped into cubes
- 1 chopped small onion
- 1 chopped leek
- 1 stalk chopped celery
- 1 peeled and chopped carrot
- 1 large garlic clove, chopped
- 1 carton single cream, 100 ml
- Olive oil
- Juice from ½ lemon

The Stock

1. 1 peeled onion, chopped into quarters
2. 1 rough chopped carrot
3. 12 black peppercorns
4. 1 tsp fennel seed
5. 1 tsp turmeric powder

6. ½ bottle white wine, medium sweet and an equal amount of water

7. Small handful parsley, rough chopped

8. Prawn shells and heads

9. 2 whole cloves

10. 4 bashed garlic cloves

11. 2 whole bay leaves

12. Juice from ½ lemon

The Croutons

- 1 small whole meal baguette, sliced thinly

- Olive oil

- ½ tsp Herbes de Provence

Instructions:

1. Peel the prawns and leave to one side

2. Make the stock by putting all of the stock ingredients into a large pan and bringing up to the boil

3. Leave to simmer for about 15 minutes, on occasion crushing the prawn heads and shells with a wooden spoon

4. Strain the stock and discard all of the solid bits

5. Poach 4 prawns lightly in the stock until they are just cooked and then remove them, leaving them to one side for garnish

6. Fry the carrot, onion, leek, and celery in some olive oil until they are soft, around 10 minutes

7. Turn the heat down and add the garlic cook for about 5 minutes

8. Add the stock and bring up to the boil

9. Add the white fish and prawns and poach for about 3 minutes

10. Remove the stock from the heat and blend it until smooth with a stick blender

11. Add the cream and season to taste

12. If serving now, keep it warm; if not cool it and refrigerate

13. Now make the croutons by frying the baguette slices in the oil until golden; drain on paper towels and sprinkle the herbs over the top

14. Serve the warm soup garnished with a prawn and a little smoked paprika and the croutons

Cauliflower Soup

Preparation time: 10 minutes

Cooking time: 30 minutes

Serves 4

Ingredients:

- Extra virgin olive oil for sautéing
- 2 large leeks, sliced finely
- 3 large celery stalks, sliced thinly
- 2 bashed garlic cloves
- 1 heaped tsp ground cumin
- 1 level tsp turmeric powder
- 1 small dried ground chili (optional)
- 1 lb. chopped cauliflower florets
- 1 medium peeled and diced potato
- 1 liter vegetable stock
- Salt and pepper for seasoning

Instructions:

1. Heat a little oil and sauté the celery and leek until soft and golden
2. Add the garlic and turn the heat down; sauté for a minute or 2, stirring
3. Add the turmeric, cumin, and the chili if using it and sauté gently, stirring, for about 1 minute

4. Add the potato and cauliflower, pour in the stock and stir

5. Season and bring to the boil; cover and simmer for 10 minutes or so, until the cauliflower and potato are cooked. Remove from the heat

6. Blend roughly with a hand blender, leaving some of the vegetable chunks whole

7. Season to tastes and serve with croutons or on its own

White Bean Soup

Preparation time: 20 minutes

Cooking time: 30 minutes

Serves 4

Ingredients:

- 1 tbsp. vegetable oil
- 1 chopped onion
- 1 chopped celery stalk
- 1 minced garlic clove
- 2 cans, 16 oz. each, white kidney beans
- 1 14 oz. can chicken broth
- ¼ tsp ground black pepper
- 1/8 tsp dried thyme
- 2 cups water
- 1 bunch fresh washed and sliced spinach
- 1 tbsp. freshly squeezed lemon juice

Instructions:

1. Heat the oil in a large pan and cook the celery and onion for about 5 to 8 minutes, or until they are soft
2. Add the garlic and cook for a further 30 seconds, stirring continually
3. Drain and rinse the beans and stir in, adding the broth, thyme, pepper, and water

4. Bring up to a boil, turn the heat down and simmer for about 15 minutes

5. Remove 2 cups of the vegetables from the soup, using a slotted spoon and set to one side

6. Blend the rest of the soup on a low speed until smooth – do it in batches if necessary

7. Pour the soup back into the pan and stir the reserved vegetables back in

8. Bring up to a boil, stirring occasionally, and then add the spinach, cooking for about a minute until the spinach has wilted

9. Stir the lemon juice in, and serve with a garnish of grated parmesan cheese

Chapter 8: Salads

Fennel Tuna and Egg Salad with Olives

Preparation time: 15 minutes

Cooking time: 5 – 10 minutes

Serves 4

Ingredients:

The Dressing:

- 1 tsp fresh lemon zest
- 1 tbsp. fresh lemon juice
- 4 tbsp. extra virgin olive oil
- 1 tsp fennel greens, chopped
- ¼ tsp salt
- Salt and pepper for seasoning

The Salad:

- 1 small peeled red onion, sliced into thin rounds
- Rice or white wine vinegar
- 1 yellow seeded pepper, veins removed and sliced thinly
- 2 small fennel bulbs, trimmed and sliced lengthways, thinly
- 8 radishes, French Breakfast variety if possible
- 12 green and black olives
- 2 hardboiled eggs, sliced into quarters

- 1 small can of tuna in water, drained
- 1 tbsp. capers

Instructions:

1. To make the dressing, combine the juice, zest, salt, oil, and ground pepper in a bowl; stir the fennel greens in

2. To make the salad, toss the slices of onion in some vinegar and leave to marinate. Turn them occasionally so that they are brightly colored.

3. Arrange the rings of pepper on a plate and top off with the fennel slices

4. Alternate the olives and radishes around the edge of the platter and place the tuna into the middle

5. Scatter the tuna with capers and arrange the egg quarters around the edge of it

6. Drain the onion and arrange over the salad

7. Spoon dressing over and serve

Greek Salad Skewers

Preparation time: 20 minutes

Cooking time: 5 minutes

Serves 4

Ingredients:

- 2 oz. cubed feta
- 2 tbsp. extra virgin olive oil
- ½ tsp dried oregano
- 1 lemon, sliced into 6 wedges
- 2 slices Italian bread, 1 inch thick and cut into 16 cubes of 1 inch
- 16 cherry tomatoes
- 1 can artichoke hearts, drained and cut in half lengthways (14 oz. can)
- ½ small red onion, peeled and chopped into 1 inch cubes
- 1 small sliced cucumber
- 20 leaves of romaine lettuce (inner leaves only)
- 12 olives, assorted, pitted

Instructions:

1. Soak 8 bamboo skewers, about 8-10 inches in water for half an hour
2. Toss the feta in oregano and oil and squeeze two of the lemon wedges over the top. Season to taste

3. Lightly oil a grill

4. Thread each bamboo skewer with alternate chunks of bread, artichoke, tomato, and onion

5. Coat with a little olive oil and grill until golden brown, turning to cook all over, about 4 minutes – do remove before the tomato falls apart.

6. Arrange the lettuce between 4 plates and top off with 2 skewers on each plate

7. Divide the feta mix between the plates

8. Divide the cucumber and olives between each plate and serve garnished with a wedge of lemon

Potato Salad, Mediterranean-Style

Preparation time: 10 minutes

Cooking time: 35-45 minutes

Serves 4

Ingredients:

- 1 tbsp. extra virgin olive oil
- 1 small thinly sliced onion
- 1 crushed garlic clove
- 1 tsp fresh or dried oregano
- ½ lb. cherry tomatoes, canned
- ¼ lb. sliced roast red pepper from a jar
- ¾ lb. new potato, sliced in half if a large one
- 3/4 oz. sliced black olives
- Handful torn fresh basil leaves

Instructions:

1. Heat the oil in a large pan and cook the onion for about 5 or 10 minutes, until softened
2. Add the oregano and the garlic and cook for a further minute
3. Add the peppers and tomatoes, season, and simmer for about 10 minutes
4. Cook the potato in salted boiling water until tender, about 10 or 15 minutes
5. Drain and mix with the sauceServe warm sprinkled with basil and olives

Fig and Mozzarella Salad

Preparation time: 5 minutes

Cooking time: 5 minutes

Serves 2

Ingredients:

- ½ lb. trimmed green beans
- 6 small fresh figs, cut into quarters
- 1 thin sliced shallot
- 1 ball of mozzarella, about 4 ½ oz., drained and torn into chunks
- 1 ¾ oz. toasted and chopped hazelnuts
- Small handful of torn fresh basil leaves
- 3 tbsp. balsamic vinegar
- 1 tbsp. fig relish or jam
- 3 tbsp. extra virgin olive oil

Instructions:

1. Blanch the beans in boiling salted water for about 2 or 3 minutes
2. Drain and rinse in cold water and drain again on kitchen paper
3. Arrange the beans on a plate and top off with the shallot, figs, hazelnuts, mozzarella, and basil

4. Put the fig jam, vinegar, and olive oil into a small-lidded jar, season, and seal. Shake well and drizzle over the salad before serving

Feta and Watermelon Salad with Fresh Crisp bread

Preparation time: 70 minutes

Cooking time: 1 hour

Serves 4

Ingredients:

The Salad

- ½ a fresh watermelon (1 ½ kg), deseeded, peeled and chopped into chunks
- ½ lb. feta cheese, cut into cubes
- A large handful of pitted black olives
- A handful of fresh flat-leaf parsley and mint leaves chopped roughly
- 1 red onion, finely sliced in rings
- Balsamic vinegar and olive oil for serving

The Crisp bread

- ½ lb. bread mix, white
- 1 tbsp. extra virgin olive oil, plus extra
- Plain flour for dusting
- 1 beaten egg white
- Fennel, poppy, and sesame seed for scattering

Instructions:

1. Make the bread mix by following the pack instructions and include 1 tbsp. olive oil in it

2. Leave it in a warm place for 1 hour to rise until it is double the size

3. In the meantime, preheat your oven to 220° F

4. Divide the risen dough into 6 equal pieces and roll out on a floured surface, as thin as possible

5. Transfer the flat dough to baking trays and brush with the beaten egg white and scatter the seeds over the top

6. Bake until brown and crisp, about 15 minutes

7. You can do this the day before if you want and store them in an airtight container until you need them

8. Toss the melon with the olives and feta and scatter the onion and herbs over the top

9. Serve on plates and drizzle the vinegar and oil over the top

10. Serve with the crisp breads

Tuscan Tuna Salad

Preparation time: 10 minutes

Serves 4

Ingredients:

- 2 cans tuna in water or oil, drained (6 oz. cans)
- 10 cherry tomatoes, cut into quarters
- 4 trimmed and sliced scallions
- 2 tbsp. extra virgin olive oil
- 2 tbsp. freshly squeezed lemon juice
- ¼ tsp salt
- 1 15 oz. can white beans, drained and rinsed
- Ground black pepper for seasoning

Instructions:

1. Mix the beans, tuna, scallions, tomatoes, lemon juice, pepper, oil, and salt together gently
2. Refrigerate until ready to use

Chapter 9: Main Courses

Tomato and Eggplant Pasta Bake

Preparation time: 15 minutes

Cooking time: 40 minutes

Serves 6

Ingredients:

- 1 lb. eggplant, cubed
- 1 lb. small tomatoes, about 2 inches in diameter, cut in half
- 1 large bell pepper, red, chopped coarsely
- 1 large onion, chopped coarsely
- 8 oz. quinoa rotelle OR whole wheat fusilli
- ¼ cup fresh basil pesto
- 4 tbsp. fresh basil, chopped
- ¼ cup parmesan, finely grated
- ¼ tsp salt
- ¼ tsp ground black pepper

Instructions:

1. Heat your broiler
2. Place the tomatoes, cut-side up, on an oiled baking tray with the eggplant, onion, and bell pepper.
3. Coat the vegetables with a little olive oil and season with the salt and pepper

4. Broil until the vegetables are tender and golden brown in color, stirring al except for the tomatoes.

5. In the meantime, heat your oven to 375° F

6. Cook the pasta as per the package instructions

7. Drain well and toss with the vegetables, the pesto and half of the fresh chopped basil

8. Spoon into an oiled shallow baking pan and top off with the cheese

9. Cover the pan with foil and bake until warmed through, about 15 or 20 minutes

10. Serve sprinkled with the rest of the fresh basil

Whole Roasted Fish with Lemon and Oregano

Preparation time: 20 minutes

Cooking time: 20 minutes

Serves 4

Ingredients:

- 1 tbsp. extra virgin olive oil
- 2 tsp freshly squeezed lemon juice
- ½ tsp dried oregano
- 1 tsp salt
- ¼ tsp ground black pepper
- 2 sliced garlic cloves
- 2 whole sea bass, cleaned
- 8 slices of lemon

Instructions:

1. Preheat your broiler or grill and oil the rack lightly
2. Whisk the oil with the juice, pepper, oregano, and half of the salt; set to one side
3. Make 3 vertical shallow slits on each side of both fish
4. Rub the rest of the salt into the fish
5. Brush the oil mixture on the inside of the fish; stuff the garlic and lemon slices inside the fish
6. Grill for about 15 to 20 minutes, turning twice and basting with the rest of the oil mixture until the fish

is a golden-brown color and the flesh has started turning opaque

7. Leave it to rest for about 10 minutes before you serve with a side salad

Greek Chicken

Preparation time: 2 hours

Cooking time: 6 minutes

Serves 4

Ingredients:

The Chicken

- 4 chicken breast halves, skinless and boneless
- 1 tbsp. freshly squeezed lemon juice
- 1 tbsp. extra virgin olive oil
- ½ tsp salt
- ¼ tsp ground black pepper
- 1 tsp dried oregano
- 1 minced garlic clove

The Yogurt

- 1 ¼ cup fat-free Greek yogurt
- ½ cup shredded cucumber
- 2 minced cloves garlic
- 1 tsp freshly chopped dill
- ½ cup pistachios, shelled and chopped coarsely

Instructions:

1. Butterfly the chicken breast. To do this, place a breast piece on a surface, shiny side facing up and with the pointed end facing you. Put your hand on the chicken

breast and, holding a knife in a parallel position to the table, push it into the thickest part of the chicken and slice almost through the chicken. Open it up like a book and gently flatten it. Repeat with the rest of the chicken

2. Mix the oil, oregano, lemon juice and garlic together and marinade the chicken in it for a couple of hours in the refrigerator. Turn the chicken occasionally

3. Put the yogurt into a coffee strainer set over a bowl and refrigerate for up to 2 hours to drain

4. Mix the yogurt with the dill, cucumber, garlic, and half of the pistachios

5. Preheat the grill

6. Take the chicken out of the marinade and sprinkle the salt and pepper over

7. Grill on an oiled grill rack for a couple of minutes on each side until cooked all the way through

8. Serve the chicken topped off with the yogurt and garnished with the rest of the pistachios

Barley Risotto with Mushrooms

Preparation time: 15 minutes

Cooking time: 35 minutes

Serves 6

Ingredients:

- 1 oz. dried mushroom
- 2 cups boiling water
- 2 cups low salt beef broth
- 2 tsp extra virgin olive oil
- 1/4 lb. sliced button mushrooms
- 1 small chopped onions
- 3 chopped garlic cloves
- 1 cup barley
- 2 tsp dried sage
- ¼ tsp salt
- ½ cup parmesan cheese, grated

Instructions:

1. Mix the dried mushrooms with the boiling water and leave it to stand for about 15 minutes
2. Place a coffee filter or some paper towels into a fine sieve and set it over a saucepan
3. Pour the steeped mushrooms through the sieve, retaining the liquid

4. Chop the mushrooms and leave to one side

5. Add the broth to the mushroom liquid and heat over a medium heat

6. Warm up the oil in a Dutch oven on a medium heat and cook all of the mushrooms, garlic, and onion for a few minutes, stirring occasionally

7. Add the sage, barley, and salt, stir, and cook for 2 minutes

8. Add a cup of the broth and cook for 5 minutes, stirring constantly – the broth should be absorbed into the mixture

9. Continue cooking and stirring for about 20 or 25 minutes, adding the broth ½ cup at a time, until the barley is tender and the liquid is absorbed

10. Serve topped with the cheese

Lemon-Turkey Cutlets

Preparation time: 10 minutes

Cooking time: 20 minutes

Serves 4

Ingredients:

- ¼ cup all-purpose flour

- 1 large egg

- 4 turkey breast cutlets, skinless and boneless, cut in half crossways

- 2 tbsp. extra virgin olive oil

- ½ lemon sliced into 8 thin slices

- 2 tbsp. pitted green olives or capers, rinsed, drained and chopped

- ½ cup dry white wine

- 1 cup low salt chicken broth

- 1 tbsp. butter unsalted variety

- ¼ tsp salt

- ¼ tsp ground black pepper

- ¼ cup flat leaf parsley, chopped – optional

Instructions:

1. Mix the flour with the salt and pepper on a shallow plate

2. Add 1 tbsp. water to the egg and beat well in a shallow bowl

3. Dredge the turkey pieces in the flour and shake the excess off

4. Dip in the egg, coating thoroughly and drip the excess off

5. Heat the oil in a large pan on a medium high heat

6. Cook the turkey for about 6 or 7 minutes, turning, until cooked through and golden brown

7. Remove the turkey from the pan and leave to one side

8. Cook the capers/olives and lemon slices in the pan until the lemon has gone a golden-brown color, around 2 minutes

9. Remove the lemon and set aside

10. Add the wine to the pan, follow with the broth and simmer for about 6 minutes, until it has thickened a little

11. Put the turkey back in the pan and stir the parsley and butter in

12. Simmer for about 5 minutes, or until the turkey is warmed through

13. Serve with the lemon slices

Scallops Provençale

Preparation time: 35 minutes

Cooking time: 50 minutes

Serves 8

Ingredients:

- 2 tbsp. unsalted butter
- 1 lb. rinsed and drained sea scallops
- 1 small finely chopped onion
- ½ lb. thin sliced mushrooms
- 1 minced garlic clove
- 2 peeled and chopped medium tomatoes
- ¼ cup dry white wine
- 2 tbsp. ketchup
- ½ tsp salt
- ½ tsp dried and chopped tarragon
- ¼ tsp dried rosemary
- Pinch of white pepper
- ¼ lb. small cooked shrimp, frozen
- 2 tsp white wine vinegar
- Fresh chopped parsley for garnish

Instructions:

1. Preheat your oven to 400° F

2. Heat the butter over a medium heat and lightly brown off the scallops – don't crowd them, cook in batches if necessary. Remove the scallops and place them in buttered baking shells or individual casserole dishes

3. Cook the mushrooms and onions in the skillet until the onion softens and starts to brown

4. Stir the tomatoes, garlic, and ketchup. Wine, salt, herbs, and white pepper in, and bring to a boil

5. Cover the pan, turn the heat down and simmer for about 15 minutes

6. Uncover and cook for a further 3 minutes or until it has thickened

7. Mix the vinegar and shrimp in and then spoon the mixture over the scallops

8. Bake until the sauce has started to bubble and has begun to brown around the edges, around 10 minutes

9. Serve garnished with parsley

Chapter 10: Desserts

Baklava

Preparation time: 20 minutes

Cooking time: 35 minutes

Makes 24 pieces

Ingredients:

- 3 cups coarsely chopped unsalted pistachio nuts
- 1/3 cup sugar
- 2 tsp fresh orange zest
- ¼ tsp ground cloves
- 1/8 tsp unsalted butter
- Cooking spray – butter flavored if you can get it
- 24 sheets phyllo pastry, 17 by 12 inch, cut in half crossways
- 1 tbsp. water
- ¾ cup organic honey
- ¼ cup fresh squeezed orange juice
- 1 tbsp. freshly squeezed lemon juice
- ½ tsp ground cardamom

Instructions:

1. Preheat your oven to 350° F

2. Put the pistachios in a bowl with the orange zest, sugar, salt, and cloves; combine well and set to one side

3. Oil a 9 by 13-inch baking dish with the spray

4. Place one sheet of phyllo length ways in the base of the dish and drape one end over the end of the dish

5. Spray lightly with cooking spray

6. Repeat with 5 more sheets

7. Sprinkle 1/3 of the nut mixture over the top

8. Repeat this procedure twice more

9. With the last nut layer, coat with 6 phyllo sheets, oiled and then oil the top sheet, pressing it down gently into the dish

10. Sprinkle a little water over the top

11. Make 6 even crossways cuts and 4 even lengthways cuts to make 24 portions

12. Bake for 30 minutes until golden brown

13. In the meanwhile, mix the lemon and orange juice, the honey, and the cardamom together over a low heat and cook for about 2 minutes or until the honey has dissolved completely

14. Drizzle over the baklava and leave to cool off completely before serving

Baked Apple

Preparation time: 10 minutes

Cooking time: 45 minutes

Serves 2

Ingredients:

- 2 large cooking apples, sharp rather than sweet
- 2 tbsp. organic honey
- ¼ tsp ground cinnamon
- ¼ tsp mixed spice
- 1 ½ oz. walnuts, roughly chopped
- 1 ½ oz. sultanas, roughly chopped
- Juice and zest of ½ lemon

Instructions:

1. Preheat your oven to 350° F
2. Use a corer or a sharp knife to remove the cores from the apples
3. Around the center of each apple, make a continuous cut, about 1/8-inch deep
4. Cut a little piece of apple from the core and push it down the center of the apple, sealing the hole at the base
5. Put both apples into a baking dish
6. Mix all the other ingredients together, combining thoroughly

7. Divide the mixture between the two apples, pushing it down firmly into the center of them and finishing with a small mound on the top

8. Pour ½ inch of water into the dish

9. Bake for about 40 or 45 minutes in the center of the oven, until the apple is golden brown and soft

10. Serve straightaway, pouring the juice over the top and adding a little crème Fraiche

Lemon Pudding

Preparation time: 5 minutes

Cooking time: 5 minutes

Serves 4

Ingredients:

- ¾ cup sugar
- ¼ cup cornstarch
- 2 ½ cups milk
- 3 egg yolks, beaten lightly
- Zest from 2 lemons
- A pinch of salt
- Juice from 2 lemons
- 2 tsp butter, unsalted
- Crushed digestive biscuits and whipped cream for decorating

Instructions:

1. Whisk the cornstarch and the sugar together
2. Add in the milk and whisk until you have a smooth consistency
3. Now whisk the salt, zest, and egg yolks in, combining thoroughly
4. Pour the mixture into a pan and heat over a medium heat, stirring constantly with a wooden spoon until the sauce is thick enough to coat the back of a spoon

5. Take the pan off the heat and stir the butter and lemon juice in

6. Divide the mixture between 4 bowls and leave to cool before covering with plastic wrap and chilling for several hours

7. Before you serve, sprinkle with crushed biscuit and whipped cream

Orange and Lemon Ricotta Cake

Preparation time: 15 minutes

Cooking time: 70 minutes

Serves 8

Ingredients:

- 3 lb. fresh ricotta cheese
- 8 whole eggs
- ½ lb. sugar
- Zest from a fresh orange
- Zest from a fresh lemon
- Butter to coat the pan

Instructions:

1. Preheat the oven to 425° F
2. Mix all of the ingredients together thoroughly in a bowl
3. Coat a 9-inch pan all over with butter
4. Pour in the mixture, coating the pan evenly
5. Bake for 30 minutes
6. Reduce the heat to 380° F and cook for a further 40 minutes
7. Cool before serving

Pavlova

Preparation time: 15 minutes

Cooking time: 3 hours

Serves 4

Ingredients:

- 7 oz. castor sugar
- 4 egg whites
- 2 tsp vinegar
- 1 tbsp. corn starch or corn flour
- 1 cup whipping cream
- 1 segmented orange
- 1 sliced kiwi
- 6 or 8 large ripe strawberries

Instructions:

1. Preheat the oven to 300° F
2. Whisk up the egg whites until stiff peaks are formed
3. Whisk the sugar in, one tbsp. at a time and then whisk in the vinegar
4. Lastly, whisk in the cornstarch
5. Line a flat baking tray with baking paper and grease it with olive oil spray
6. Put the meringue mix onto the paper in a 10-inch circle. It should be 3 ½ inches deep

7. Put the meringue into the middle of the oven, shut the door and immediately reduce the heat to 245° F

8. Cook for about 2 ½ to 3 hours until the meringue is a creamy color and crisp to touch

9. Turn off the oven and leave the meringue to cool down totally

10. When cold, peel the greaseproof paper off

11. Place the pavlova on a plate and pile on thickly whipped cream, spreading it over the top almost to the edge

12. Decorate using fruits of your choice

Tuscan Grape Cake

Preparation time: 10 minutes

Cooking time: 45 minutes

Serves 12

Ingredients:

- ¾ cup all-purpose flour
- ½ cup ground almond
- ½ cup corn meal
- 2 tsp baking powder
- ½ tsp salt
- 1/3 cup vegetable oil
- ¾ cup brown sugar, light variety
- 1 tsp almond extract
- 3 eggs
- ½ cup sour cream
- 2 cups seedless red grapes
- 1 tbsp. brown sugar
- 1 tbsp. white sugar

Instructions:

1. Preheat the oven to 350° F
2. Blend the almonds, flour, salt, baking powder and cornmeal together

3. In another bowl, mix together the light brown sugar, almond extract, and the oil

4. Add in the eggs, beating them in one at a time

5. Add the cream, whisking to combine

6. Add the flour mixture in and combine well

7. Grease a 9-inch springform pan and pour the mixture in evenly

8. Bake for 10 minutes

9. Remove the cake from the oven and spread the grapes in an even layer over the top

10. Mix together the brown and white sugars, sprinkle over the top and bake for a further 30 to 35 minutes

11. Leave to cool completely before cutting to serve

Chapter 11: Snacks

Marinated Olives with Feta Cheese

Preparation time: 70 minutes

Serves 12

Ingredients:

- 1 cup of olives, pitted and sliced
- ½ cup feta cheese, diced
- 2 tbsp. extra virgin olive oil
- Juice and zest of one lemon
- 2 sliced garlic cloves
- 1 tsp fresh chopped rosemary
- Fresh ground black pepper for seasoning
- Pinch of crushed red pepper

Instructions:

1. Combine all of the ingredients together in a bowl
2. Cover the bowl and refrigerate for 24 hours before serving

Hummus

Preparation time: 5 minutes

Serves 4

Ingredients:

- 1 16 oz. can rinsed and drained chickpeas
- 1/3 cup fat-free plain yogurt
- ¼ cup scallions, minced
- ¼ cup finely minced fresh parsley
- Juice from 2 lemons
- 5 tsp tahini
- 1 tbsp. olive oil
- 3 minced garlic cloves
- 1/8 tsp ground black pepper
- Low salt soy sauce
- Ground red pepper

Instructions:

1. Put the chickpeas in a blender and blend until smooth
2. Scrape the sides occasionally to make sure it is all combined
3. Add the scallions, yogurt, parsley, tahini, juice, garlic, oil, black pepper, and a splash of soy sauce
4. Process until you have a smooth creamy consistency – add a little water if needed

5. Spoon into a serving bowl, sprinkle red pepper and serve with crudités for dipping

Cherries with Ricotta & Toasted Almonds

Preparation time: 5 minutes

Cooking time: 1-2 minutes

Serves 1

Ingredients:

- ¾ cup pitted cherries, frozen
- 2 tbsp. ricotta, part-skim
- 1 tbsp. slivered toasted almonds

Instructions:

1. Warm the cherries in a bowl in the microwave for a couple of minutes
2. Layer the cherries in a bowl and top off with the ricotta and almonds

Tomato & Basil Finger Sandwiches

Preparation time: 5 minutes

Serves 4

Ingredients:

- 4 slices bread, whole grain
- 8 tsp mayonnaise, low-fat
- 4 thick tomato slices
- 4 tsp fresh sliced basil
- 1/8 tsp salt
- 1/8 tsp. ground black pepper

Instructions:

1. Cut rounds from the bread that are a little larger than your tomato slices
2. Spread mayonnaise over each slice
3. Layer the tomato and basil on top and season with salt and pepper

Date Wraps

Preparation time: 10 minutes

Serves 4

Ingredients:

- 16 whole dates, pitted
- 16 prosciutto slices
- Ground pepper for seasoning

Instructions:

1. Wrap each date in a slice of prosciutto
2. Season with pepper

Blueberries with Lemon Cream

Preparation time: 10 minutes

Serves 4

Ingredients:

- 4 oz. cream cheese, low fat
- ¾ cup vanilla yogurt, low fat
- 1 tsp honey
- 2 tsp lemon zest
- 2 cups fresh blueberries

Instructions:

1. Break the cream cheese up in a bowl, using a fork
2. Drain the yogurt to discard any excess liquid and add the yogurt and the honey to the cream cheese
3. Beat with an electric mixer until creamy and light
4. Stir the lemon zest in
5. Layer the cream and the blueberries in dessert dishes and, if not eating straight away, cover and cool in the refrigerator for about 8 hour

Conclusion

Thank you again for purchasing this book!

I hope this book was able to help you to understand the underlying principles of the Mediterranean diet and how it can help you to lose weight and keep it off for good. The Mediterranean diet is a healthy one and is full of fresh, whole foods and wonderful, easy to prepare recipes that you can enjoy with abandon, without having to worry about becoming obsessed with counting calories. The very nature of the diet means that you will find it easier to lose the excess pounds and feel great while you are doing it. Not all of the recipes are straightforward but most of them are simple to prepare and cook and the effort will most definitely be worthwhile.

The next step is to, quite simply, start the diet! Make your shopping list from the list of foods provided for you and head off to the store. Like any diet, you may find it difficult to change your eating habits but, once you get into it, you will find it easy to stick to and follow. Change your life today; lose weight, and improve your health and energy levels no end by taking up the challenge of the Mediterranean diet a new lifestyle, a new you.

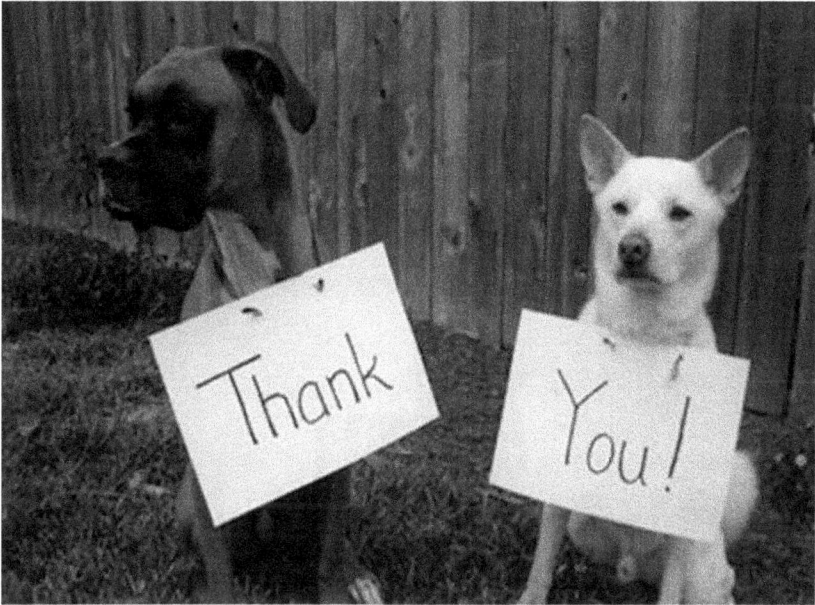

Finally, if you enjoyed this book, then I'd like to ask you for a favor, would you be kind enough to leave a review for this book on Amazon? It'd be greatly appreciated!

Click here to leave a review for this book on Amazon!

Thank you and good luck with your journey to a new, healthy you!

Check Out Our Other Books

Below you'll find some of my other popular books that are popular on Amazon and Kindle as well. Simply click on the links below to check them out. Alternatively, you can visit my author page on Amazon to see other work done by me.

Muscle Building: Beginners Handbook - Proven Step By Step Guide To Get The Body You Always Dreamed About

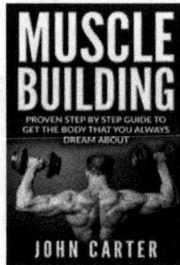

www.ingramcontent.com/pod-product-compliance
Lightning Source LLC
Chambersburg PA
CBHW071243020426
42333CB00015B/1598